My Father's Journey with Dementia

Pamela Kida

Copyright © 2020 Pamela Kida

Healing Hearts and Families Press— Glen Allen, VA
ISBN: 978-0-578-68607-3
Library of Congress Control Number: pending
Title: My Father's Journey with Dementia
Author: Pamela Kida
Digital distribution | 2020
Paperback | 2020

Dedication

I dedicate this book to my mother who is a source of inspiration and strength for having the perseverance and love in caring for Dad throughout his life. To the Deli Girls, a loving group of women who continue to support each other during the most stressful times of their lives. To my family, mom, sister, and brother in recognition of our loss. To my husband and my children for being my sounding board, helping and supporting me through the loss of my father. I dedicate this book to the memories of our loved ones who we have lost to this disease. Finally, I dedicate this book to my Dad, I miss you and you will forever be in our hearts.

For more information, please visit the Alzheimer's organization's website http://www.alz.org/. For a support group, please join us on Facebook: The Deli Girls. The Deli Girls support group is an online, private Facebook page where you can share your story.

Table of Contents

Abstract

Experiencing the loss of a loved one is difficult. Grief brings on many different emotions and even contradictory feelings such as relief, remorse, sadness, anger and more. For me it has brought on a determination in finding ways to memorialize my father and to raise awareness of Alzheimer's disease.

After Dad's death, I searched for grief support groups but I didn't feel comfortable meeting and sharing my grief at the age of 61 years old. At this age, there is a natural cycle of life and having your parents pass away is part of that cycle. I had recently experienced the loss of my Uncle Bill who died of Alzheimer's four years earlier, in 2014, and now my father. I'm 61 and wondering if this day to day experience of losing my glasses, misplacing my car keys and not finding the tv remote is symptomatic of the disease? Will I also fall victim to Alzheimer's? Will I develop the rare blood disease akin to leukemia like my father did? I can accept my father's passing he was fortunate to live a long life, fairly peacefully even with Type 1 diabetes and dementia. I discovered things about my Dad, his soft-hearted soul and gentleness because of the onset of dementia.

In the early days of Dad's dementia, Mom signed Dad up for Adult Day Care. A wonderful place where Dad could stay for the day, be involved in activities specifically designed for elder care support.

This is where Mom met a lady involved in a support group, affectionately known as 'The Deli Girls', a women's support group whose husband's were diagnosed with Alzheimer's. The Deli Girls were the primary caretakers for their husbands diagnosed with some form of dementia. This group formed in the year 2010 and since then, they have met every Friday for lunch at the local deli. Thus begins the story of my father's journey with dementia, my mother's journey as the primary caretaker and "The Deli Girls" and how I came to know them.

Acknowledgments

It is with sincere gratitude to all the ladies who make up The Deli Girls group, whose support they have given to my mother, I cannot thank enough. It is because of the special bond these ladies have, that propelled me to share my story about Dementia from a daughter's perspective.

To my friends and to the people who I have met along the way who had the willingness to share information, contacts, and pearls of wisdom to make this book happen.

To my friends who supported the efforts in writing this book and to Richard DiGiacomo, author of '*The Day Julie Brought Her Lion* to School', who helped direct the success of this book by recommending New Book Authors (www.newbookauthors.com).

Preface

When embarking on this project, a group of women whose husbands had been diagnosed with Alzheimer's, provided support with a purpose to raise awareness about Alzheimer's (http://www.alz.org/). Do you know someone who is suffering from dementia, maybe Alzheimer's? This disease is slow to develop and the deterioration of the brain does not happen overnight. When the going gets rough – you have to search for those shining moments that do exist, just not in the way that you were expecting. As you can tell, the walk with dementia and Alzheimer's is not for the faint of heart. It is a journey of fear, anger, sadness, acceptance, and relief. Everyone's journey is different just as the effects of dementia are different for each person. However, the trajectory and finality of Alzheimer's are the same – it robs the person of their memories, past and present, and it is their last journey on this earth.

President Ronald Reagan's Letter

"Nov. 5, 1994
  My Fellow Americans,

I have recently been told that I am one of the millions of Americans who will be afflicted with Alzheimer's Disease.

Upon Learning this news, Nancy and I had to decide whether as private citizens we would keep this a private matter or whether we would make this news known in a public way.

In the past Nancy suffered from breast cancer and I had my cancer surgeries. We found through our open disclosures we were able to raise public awareness. We were happy that as a result many more people underwent testing.

They were treated in early stages and able to return to normal, healthy lives.
  So now, we feel it is important to share it with you. In opening our hearts, we hope this might promote greater awareness of this condition. Perhaps it will encourage a clearer understanding of the individuals and families who are affected by it.

At the moment I feel just fine. I intend to live the remainder of the years God gives me on this earth doing the things I have always done. I will continue to share life's journey with my beloved Nancy and my family. I plan to enjoy the great outdoors and stay in touch with my friends and supporters.

Unfortunately, as Alzheimer's Disease progresses, the family often bears a heavy burden. I only wish there was some way I could spare Nancy from this painful experience. When the times comes I am confident that with your help she will face it with faith and courage.

In closing let me thank you, the American people for giving me the great honor of allowing me to serve as your President. When the Lord calls me home, whenever that may be, I will leave with the greatest love for this country of ours and eternal optimism for its future.

I now begin the journey that will lead me into the sunset of my life. I know that for America there will always be a bright dawn ahead.

Thank you, my friends. May God always bless you.
    Sincerely,
    Ronald Reagan"
    (Reagan, 1994)

In the Beginning…In the End

My father was a conservative man born in 1928 in the deep south of Macon, Georgia. Growing up, Dad moved from Macon, Georgia, to San Antonio, Texas, then Newport News, Virginia. While in High School, he was awarded a full scholarship to the college of William and Mary, a research University in Williamsburg, Virginia where he received his Bachelor of Science. He then moved to New York City to attend Columbia University where he received his Masters in Public Health Administration. He lived in New York City while building his career (and yes, he went on a date with one of the Radio City Music Hall Rockettes!). While living in New York City, he met the love of his life at a party, my mother, Audrey Jean Fenton. They married December 5, 1952, in Jackson Heights, Queens.

My mother is a very talented pianist and artist. At the age of 19, she was accepted into Julliard and instead of enrolling in Julliard, she pursued her teaching degree and became a successful teacher, retiring after a 32-year career. This becomes important because it requires an enormous amount of courage, strength, and perseverance when one becomes the caretaker, "... in sickness and in health, until death do us part'.

After his retirement, Dad founded a senior professional consulting group aptly named "The Professional Group" at George Mason University in Fairfax, Virginia. As he got older, and after the dementia had started to really kick in, Dad attended the Lincolnia Senior Center, an adult daycare. My Dad could be very funny at times and throughout his entire life, enjoyed being social. However, when the Dementia started, where he could realize something wasn't right, he started to withdraw.

My mother and father had three children, Susan (1954), David (1956) and myself (Pam, 1958). It was early enough in my parent's marriage that Dad's Diabetes did not yet interfere with life too much where mom and dad could give their attention to family life. They raised three children who married and raised children of their own: Susan (Scott), David, Pamela (John) and gave Mom and Dad eight very special grand-children (Benjamin, Jeffrey, Caleigh, Brian, Katelyn, Jeffrey, Mark, and Jordanka).

My sister, the oldest of the three kids, was smart in school, she was motivated and had high aspirations for herself. She grew up to be a dentist married her husband, also a dentist, and has three grown children. My sister's oldest son, Ben, would call Grandma and Grandpa from California (we live in Virginia) just to say Hello! This still brings a smile to my face because those calls meant a lot to them – it made them happy. Trust me, when you are facing your senior years, you start counting on all those things that make you smile. Susan continues to share her talents and volunteers her time with the local Rotary and with the World Dental Health Organization. She has traveled to both Honduras and Kenya in her volunteer efforts.

My brother is the middle child, graduated from William and Mary with a degree in Marine Biology, subsequently receiving his Masters and continuing his research for the Commonwealth of Virginia. David has a family with two grown children living in Virginia.

My name is Pam and I am the youngest, married with three grown children. I graduated from the University of Richmond (Business) and Liberty University (M.Ed.). I retired after 38 years with the Commonwealth of Virginia from a career in Information Technology, IT Project Management. Retirement provides me the freedom to write and to care for Mom now that Dad has passed.

The grandkids all took a level of interest in their grandparents. Ben took Grandpa jet skiing on the lake with Grandpa dressed in his khakis and dress shoes. It was a great memory. Katelyn would take Grandpa walking and get his leg muscles moving. My stepson, Jeffrey, and Grandpa had a special relationship because they would spend many hours conversing about anything and everything. Brian, who is a firefighter, would call and check in on them which was very reassuring. The others would call and touch base when they could. Sometimes I would call my own kids and ask that they call Grandma and Grandpa. The grandkids are so busy, that asking that they call and say 'hello' can mean so much.

Growing up was not easy because of the chaos surrounding Dad's diabetes, but I can pick out fun times such as going to the World's Fair in Flushing, NY (1964) and baking apple pies with Dad using the apples from our Apple tree. Visiting my paternal grandparents consisted of driving in the hot summers, without air-conditioning in a big station wagon to Newport News, Virginia (where they lived in the 1960s). In the hot summers, Grandpa would take us fishing, we would catch and eat fried catfish with boiled okra. We would run to the shed in the back yard and grab bottled Coca-Cola™, then we would run and climb the big pecan tree located outside of their kitchen window. I remember to this day when Dad and a friend of his were part of a talent show at my school where Dad played the clairvoyant partner. I was certainly amazed but then I was in elementary school at that time.

Some of the dynamics in our family started to change for us kids as we grew up. I believe it to have been affected by many things that we just did not have control of. My hearing loss is defined as moderately severe due to early age earaches and a penicillin allergy. I didn't get a hearing aid until I was 25 years old. I could not tell you why I did not get a hearing aid earlier but it just didn't happen. I didn't know what I was missing until I got that hearing aid. This is an important point, because I didn't understand why people didn't perceive me as 'smart' or thought I was 'mean' because they thought I was ignoring them.

I did not understand what was happening to Dad when the ambulance arrived every week because of his low blood sugars due to Diabetes. One of Dad's remarkable strengths is that he lived with Type 1 diabetes for 77 years. He received a medal from the Joselin Center for Diabetes for his courageous efforts in living with this disease.

I inherited much from my father's side of the family including insulin dependent diabetes meaning my pancreas is not producing any insulin! It is my hope that I do not inherit Alzheimer's. I recently read an article addressing the question of Alzheimer's and inheritance, and the article indicated "…we have now learned that susceptibility to a disease may be influenced by the presence of one or more genes related less directly to the disease itself." (Ellison, 2019). Since my Uncle died from Alzheimer's and my father died of complications from Dementia, then it would be wise for me to prepare for my elder years. So far I invested in a Long Term Care policy, and picked out a couple of Assisted Living places that could handle a client with Diabetes. If I am fortunate enough, I will be able to live out my life at home.

My Dad's chronic health issues with Diabetes contributed to his disease with dementia. He was ultimately diagnosed with Vascular Dementia which is a narrowing of blood vessels in his brain. Vascular Dementia is a decline in thinking skills caused by conditions that block or reduce blood flow to various regions of the brain, depriving them of oxygen and nutrients (www.alz.org, 2019). Inadequate blood flow can damage and eventually kill cells anywhere in the body, but the brain is especially vulnerable.

In Vascular Dementia, changes in thinking skills can sometimes occur suddenly after a stroke, which blocks major blood vessels in the brain. Thinking difficulties may also begin as mild changes that gradually worsen as a result of multiple minor strokes or another condition that affects smaller blood vessels, leading to widespread damage. A growing number of experts prefer the term "Vascular Cognitive Impairment" (VCI) to "Vascular Dementia" because they feel it better expresses the concept that vascular thinking changes can range from mild to severe. Vascular brain changes often coexist with changes linked to other types of dementia, including Alzheimer's disease and Vascular Dementia.

As I watched Dad's own health decline, I couldn't help but think of my Uncle Bill who was in a nursing home in Florida. He was diagnosed with Alzheimer's and eventually died from the disease. What he had, Alzheimer's, was different than what my Dad had which was Vascular Dementia, but the symptoms and progression of the disease were very similar. During my research, I discovered that many illnesses lead to some form of dementia: Vascular Dementia, Alzheimer's, Lewy Body dementia, Parkinson's disease dementia and others where the disease affects the blood flow to the brain.

(https://www.goldencarers.com/what-is-dementia-alzheimers-disease-vs-dementia/4054/)

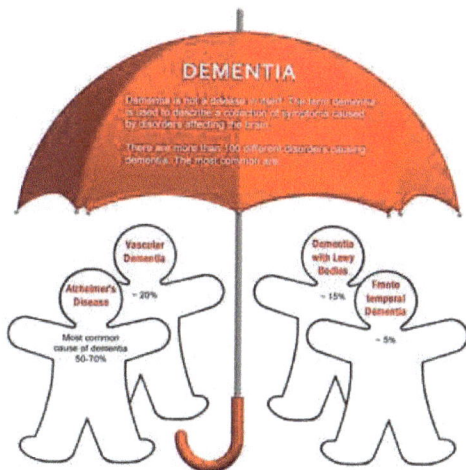

Dad could be pretty cool and a fun father but he could also be pretty rough to live with sometimes. He would bake apple pies with us kids, participate in school activities, and he even built a go-cart with my brother for a town go-cart race. That was pretty exciting. Other times, he would be angry and yell at us, when sometimes we didn't know why.

Dad would let his anger escalate over things I didn't understand and it became very bewildering. Part of the anger was because of his Diabetes, and part of that was frustration over things he didn't have control over which we believe to be a part of the Vascular Dementia. Dementia must have been slowly but surely creeping into my Dad's life for years. One day I was up visiting my parents and it was in the year 2008. Dad was standing in the kitchen, looking somewhat flustered and I looked at him, and asked what was wrong. He just looked at me and in an exasperated tone stated: "I don't know what is wrong with me, I just feel so confused!". All I could think of to say in response was "Don't worry Dad, we will take care of you." I was scared for him and afraid to have an in-depth discussion about what was happening. We all knew by then that there was something wrong, more than just forgetting. This was dementia. I didn't watch the movie featuring Nick Nolte in 'Head Full of Honey' (2018) until after Dad's passing, but when I did see it, I finally understood the depth of what Dad was saying.

A lesson I learned from this experience would be to face the fear head on. Find the support groups, consult with an eldercare specialist who can help treat the disease and manage the symptoms. It is better to pre-empt the disease so you already have the tools in your toolbox. To be unprepared makes it that much harder on the caretaker, if not near impossible to properly manage the situation. We did not always pre-empt the different situations encountered but mom was phenomenal in what she did and it was because of her support group, The Deli Girls, that helped her through it.

At this point in time, my mother was retired from full-time teaching but was still substituting. Suddenly, my mother stopped substitute teaching after 32 years because she needed to stay home and care for Dad. His dementia grew into something much more than forgetfulness.

Dad required help in the morning to just get out of bed. He needed help in eating his meals, managing his insulin, taking his shots, and taking his pills. Dad continued to stay home, look at the newspaper, and putter around. Unbeknown to anyone, he was out collecting – coins, stamps, pictures. I wish he shared it with us – I found it fascinating because he was interested in these things. The collections were not worth much money which we found out after his death but they were a part of him. We didn't know when he started, how long he was collecting for or how much he spent on his collection.

Eventually, my father could not remember that we went out to dinner the night before or what we talked about 5 minutes ago or in the more advance stages of the disease, one second ago. I was blessed that he always knew and remembered my mother and the family. It doesn't always happen that way. Only once did Dad ask me who I was. It was late in the evening, and I just popped into the family room and I think I just startled him. In that moment, I just looked at mom, turned around and left the room. I just did not know what to do or how to react but I was again, scared. I am thankful that it never happened again.

Whenever we entered the house, he would smile and say 'Hello' and gave him the hug that he always got! I could see near the end stages of the disease that Dad was physically declining. He could still talk, but he wanted to sleep more. Dad had other life long physical ailments besides dementia and lifelong Type 1 Diabetes. At the age of 80, he had a heart attack. Once he was stabilized, they found that he needed bypass surgery. The first group of doctors to evaluate him and his heart condition wouldn't approve of heart surgery because of his age and his medical ailments.

Dad was really struggling at that time because of his heart condition. Some doctors will do that, choose to do nothing because of high risk situations such as advanced age and chronic diseases like Diabetes. Thanks to my mother's perseverance, she found a cardiologist who would do the surgery. The doctor agreed to do the surgery and not use the bypass machine (which has known side effects on the brain) unless he had to. Dad had a double bypass at the age of 80. The surgery was very successful but recovery had its challenges. I understood now why the other doctors were so hesitant to do the surgery on Dad. He was at high risk because of his dementia and diabetes, but even more so, success hinged upon whether or not a patient with dementia could follow the after surgery therapeutic processes. We had to monitor his care 24/7 by monitoring his diabetes, his meals and his therapeutic regime. We were there to make sure success happened but I can't say that Dad was a cooperative patient. He wanted to sleep, he did not want to hold a pillow and cough, or walk, or otherwise do what was necessary to support recovery from bypass surgery. For a person with dementia, being cooperative is not the first thing that they care about.

When Dad slept, was when mom would leave the house and go shopping for groceries and just get out for a bit. One day, mom came home only to find Dad scurrying back to bed with some type of 'guilty' look on his face. The fire extinguisher had been activated with this white 'stuff' all over the kitchen counters and floors. When Mom asked what happened, his response was 'I don't know what happened.' The reality is, he really didn't know.

When mom found out about The Deli Girls, a group of 14 women whose husbands were diagnosed with Alzheimer's, was when she got her greatest support. They met every Friday at the local deli for lunch so they could spend a couple of hours together. It was a time to share their feelings, information on the latest Alzheimer's research, contact information for caretakers and doctors. This was an opportunity for these women to share their stories. There was a seriousness within the group but at the same time, there was a lot of laughter and many tears. Mom would always tell me she was going to have lunch this Friday with the girls, The Deli Girls.

I would call my mother every day and Dad was usually sleeping. When he wasn't sleeping, Mom would put Dad on the phone so I could say "Hello" and "How are you" to him. I would always ask him what he has been doing lately and he would normally respond "Ohhhh, nothing much." During these times Dad sounded pretty happy. He was able to maintain his hygiene, and maintain toiletry needs. He just couldn't remember that he had Diabetes and to take his medicines much less eat. He just wanted to take naps. His life really came alive around dinner time until 10 to 11:00 at night. He had turned into a sort of night owl.

My father was a "happy" patient with vascular dementia. Dad was on medication to help manage his mood swings. He did not necessarily go crazy and have violent tantrums, although I have heard stories that can bear testimony to the more violent tantrums in the world of Alzheimer's. For us, it wasn't crazy like that but it did become more awful near the end with Dad wanting to know what was wrong with him. We stayed in constant contact with his doctor. Dad started complaining of feeling very sick, which translated into complications with his health as the disease continued to grab hold of him. When he was able to sleep, we were all thankful. Knowing Dad was sleeping comfortably, gave us all a rest and provided comfort knowing he was O.K. at the moment. On the other hand, Dad was sleeping 14 or more hours a day! This is a sign that the disease has progressed and Dad's time with us is getting shorter and shorter.

I didn't know how bad things had gotten until much later on. Mom called and asked if I could stay with Dad while she went away for the weekend. This one time she was traveling to see my sister and my daughter was flying with her. I completely enjoyed my weekend with Dad. The shocking part was I took Dad out to an Italian restaurant, just me and him, father and daughter night out. We had a good time, he talked and reminisced about when he was growing up – it was a delightfully, warm time-sharing dinner with Dad. The next morning, he did not have any memory of going out to dinner the night before. Yes, I was shocked and there is no way to minimize that. I told myself that I couldn't dwell on the fact that he didn't remember. Instead, I shared in Dad's good mood that morning. I can't stress enough the importance of appreciating good moods. Although he may not remember specifically having dinner with me the night before, I would like to think the feelings of happiness from that time would flow into the next day.

My mother had the opportunity to travel with her older brother on a land and sea cruise to Alaska. So Dad came to stay with my husband and I for a couple of weeks. While on the cruise, Mom became sick and developed sepsis, ending up in the hospital in Juneau, Alaska. It was such a frightening time. Mom was hallucinating and didn't know really where she was because of the sepsis. The wonderful doctors and nurses in Juneau did a great job caring for my mother and for their constant communications with us. Although we told Dad what was happening with mom in Juneau, Alaska, Dad couldn't remember. We told him multiple times and even though we told him, he would get so upset and ask why we didn't tell him. Finally, Mom was escorted home with a nurse because she was on oxygen while flying home. That night, Mom and Dad both leaned into each other, happy to be together and watching television. I can unequivocally state that Dad did not remember that mom had a very close call while in Alaska.

When my Uncle died from Alzheimer's, we didn't know what or how to tell Dad. It was problematic because you could tell him, but he won't remember. So, the right thing to do was to tell him that his brother had passed. He was of course upset, became stoic, but not too long after, he was back to his old self. Mom indicated that Dad did ask about him sometime after, where mom had to tell him again that he passed. It's hard to say what he remembered.

Another time, in the later stages of the disease, Dad was beginning to have trouble making it to the bathroom on time. I am his daughter. The caretaker, Kingsly, was off for the weekend because supposedly I could handle it all. This was almost beyond my capability but I found out very quickly that it wasn't. I had to take care of Dad. What made me feel bad was he felt so apologetic when he didn't make it to the bathroom on time, or he dropped something, or fell onto the couch, he would say to me "I don't know why this happened!". We do the best we can and move on. Kingsley came back the next day – Thankfully!

How did Kingsley come into my father's life? Through the Deli Girls. Kingsley is from Ghana. His livelihood is eldercare, caring for men with dementia/Alzheimer's. One day while with The Deli Girls, mom said she had to get someone to help her because she couldn't do it herself. She didn't just want anybody and preferred a male. One of the Deli Girls then introduced Kingsley to mom.

I searched for eldercare services all over Fairfax County, Virginia and contacted the Virginia Department for Aging and Rehabilitative (DARS) services, Area Agencies for Aging (AAA) as well as the Community Services Board (CSB) of Fairfax County. Most of the services available were to those on Medicaid or were fee-based services meaning you had to be below a certain income level to qualify. Unless we had veteran benefits or other financial benefits, all you had left was to private pay for all services. The three of us did the best we could in sending Mom money to help pay for private pay services but it got expensive fast. Kingsley worked with us through all of that. During Dad's last months, last weeks, last days and last moments – Kingsley was there for us.

I was able to telecommute with my job and stay with my parents to the end when Dad passed away. The support of my co-workers were undeniable and comforting. It is so important that when you are the primary caretaker, that you find comfort by talking with others, finding volunteers, sharing with your neighbors. They will watch out for you and will be there in the time of need – at least ours were.

As time went on, at the age of 89, Dad continued to decline, more and more. Dad would develop Urinary Tract Infections (UTI) which could become septic to his body. He became very forgetful and paranoid. He was convinced that no one tested his sugar and he needed insulin. As Dad continued to feel worse, he thought that he was having an insulin reaction (a low blood sugar). I believed that Dad felt bad, but it wasn't from a low or high blood sugar because we tested his sugars routinely. Sometimes Dad's paranoia lasted 24 hours a day and the night times were the most difficult. Those times were scary and more than once, we ended up in the emergency room and they admitted him into the hospital. One time when Dad was in the hospital, he called my husband at work. He said to John, "Everyone has left me, I am alone in the hospital and I've been abandoned.". It was a very sad and poignant moment. Thankfully my husband handled it in a way that I thought was very caring and supportive by telling him that no one has abandoned you, we all love you. One of the last times we were in the emergency room and they admitted Dad into the hospital, we found out that his 'craziness' was due to low salt. Once we gave him salt pills. he was more comfortable and the up/down behaviors leveled out. There were a lot of 'this time' moments. It is part of the progression of the disease and you never know when that next time will appear and you never know how it will manifest itself. My lesson learned during this time, is to trust the doctors and the nurses. At the same time, continue to persevere in getting the necessary treatment to make the patient comfortable. There is no reason to suffer – you or them.

When you have someone in your life who needs 24/7 care, there are decisions that need to be made and none of them are easy decisions to make. We could not afford to move Dad into a nursing facility and by default, the decision was made to keep Dad at home as long as possible. There were many challenges with keeping Dad at home. One was you couldn't leave the house and leave Dad home alone.

Arrangements had to be made for in-home care. Although we called the county Community Services Board (CSB) for assistance, all their services were income-based qualifications. The CSB offered once a month respite care but we did not take advantage of it because Dad needed additional care related to his diabetes. Dad could not clearly communicate with us how he was feeling or if he was having a low blood sugar. Since mom and I were the most experienced, it fell on us to monitor and care for Dad with very little respite. Even if we could afford to put Dad in a memory care facility, he was too high of a risk with his diabetes. Some of the family wanted both parents to go into Assisted Living. It's a hard choice, one that has to be researched and well thought out. Ultimately it was up to our parents. Since Mom and Dad had a one-story home with a downstairs family room and basement, it made sense to keep Dad at home. This was a decision that we never regretted.

Whether or not to keep your loved one at home who has Alzheimer's or other dementia related disease, it is important to have a plan in place that has been discussed with the family. It is known that changing the surroundings of the Alzheimer's patient can bring about more confusion until the patient can adjust to their new surroundings. It might bring more peace to the family if one can keep the patient at home and utilize the services of a caretaker. On the other hand, if you have the resources to have your loved one cared for in a nursing home facility with a memory care unit, it might be the better choice for you and your loved one. There is no concrete rule or formula on what you should do. When we were in the process of deciding what to do, I researched private hospice/nursing homes, memory care and assisted living facilities. We also utilized a service, 'A Place for Mom' founded in 2000, a privately held, for-profit senior care referral service based in Seattle, Washington. The company provides personal and professional assistance to families in the search of senior care options (www.aplaceformom.com, 2020). I am just personally glad that we were able to keep Dad at home.

The last few weeks of Dad's life continued to be very difficult. Dad might have been having a few challenges but he was able to get out of bed and take care of his hygiene for the most part. He was cooperative in his insulin regime and be a part of our conversations. The things we had to do included hiding his insulin and syringes because he would forget that we gave him his medicines, made sure he ate, and involved him in adult daycare when we could. Then all of a sudden, things changed dramatically. He didn't feel well at all. He would call out every 2-3 minutes that he needed juice. He thought he was having an insulin reaction. This makes sense to me because he was feeling awful and that's all he knew as the cause. I would go in and talk to him and let him know that his sugar levels tested fine. I would ask him if he was feeling bad and in that second, he would say he was O.K. Then it would start all over again until we gave him an anti-anxiety pill to calm him and to help him fall asleep. Mom started setting up another round of doctor's appointments.

This time they found something in his blood that was more than just Dementia. After weeks of testing, Mom went to the specialist and found out that Dad had a rare form of cancer of the blood, a rare form of Leukemia. They thought he had a month. This is when Dad was put on Hospice and we still kept him home. The disease of Alzheimer's has debilitating effects on the body. Your brain can no longer keep your body functioning. At some point, organ failures begin and the process takes up different forms of presentation. In Dad's case, it began with dementia, confusion then physical ailments. Finally, the blood disease is yet another manifestation of his body not being able to keep healthy.

During this time, we received the hospice kit which included morphine. The Deli Girls updated the telephone tree and continued to stay in touch with Mom especially when she couldn't make it to their Friday lunch. Dad went from standing and talking to barely being able to use a walker and not being able to move by himself. He would ask what was wrong with him and I had to leave that disclosure up to Mom. She couldn't tell him he was dying from cancer. Dad was also experiencing paranoia, again. It was terrible to think how much distress he was feeling. Dad couldn't retain any information at this point and so we continued to support and comfort him the best we could. Although he was on hospice, he was suffering but still coherent. There was one time where no one was around to help us, so we called 9-1-1 and took him to the emergency room to get fluids. Although his time on earth was coming to an end, it was the best thing we could have done. Dad was much better, he looked better, and evidently felt better. We believed in comfort care and maintaining as normal of a care routine as possible. The hospice nurse at the time suggested we withhold medications including insulin and withhold water. I didn't think we needed to hurry along the death process and I thought that was just cruel. True story.

Hospice care is for those that are dying and the person's death is near. Hospice is generally for short-term care. However, a person can go on Hospice care and fall out of it (because they get better). We had that happen twice but no one could really explain the process of Hospice appropriately to us and of course, we were just concerned for Dad. It got to the point that when he went on Hospice this last time, I was very upset with the hospice nurse because of how she described Dad's care should be. Thankfully Mom and I were on the same page. We continued care and calling the hospital to get him fluids up until the last week. I think you can tell when enough is enough. When Dad was coherent (up until the last day) we continued to provide care. When the last night came, it was so evident that his body was shutting down. All care had to be done in coordination with the medical professionals. It is O.K. to question and disagree – but always consult with the medical professional.

From the time of the blood disease diagnosis, Dad lived 10 days. I was in the bedroom watching Dad sleep. The crisis from the night before required us to call the hospice nurse because Dad was really struggling. This beautiful lady (the on-call hospice nurse) came in the middle of the night, gave Dad the morphine and within 15 minutes she was able to get Dad in a comfortable place where he could sleep. Dad was dying. It was during this time, he was aware of his surroundings, but he was still sleeping. I was there when he took his last breath at 8:35AM, November 23, 2018. He was at peace. Since hospice gave us the process of what to do earlier, we were able to follow the steps to take care of Dad on his final rest.

The night the hospice nurse came to administer morphine, she advised us that this was the end that he probably wouldn't make it to the morning. My husband called the funeral home to update them on what was happening. In case you didn't know, the funeral home has an on-call person 24/7. Mom and

Dad had made prior funeral arrangements and we already knew what we had to do. It does bring a certain amount of comfort during a time of chaos. I recommend that you get familiar with a pamphlet about your final wishes. It is the first living will that talks about your personal, emotional and spiritual needs as well as your medical wishes.

We contacted the hospice nurse who then arrived to check Dad's vitals and to record the death. We contacted the funeral home to have them retrieve the body. The funeral home already had his final wishes. Even with all of that, it took hours before they finally took the body to the funeral home. That was probably the most difficult time – the wait and knowing that Dad had passed away, resting in the next room.

Since mom and dad had already made arrangements with the funeral home, our next steps were to meet with the funeral director, finalize the funeral in accordance to his wishes. We notified family and friends, and made beautiful arrangements with a local restaurant for us to gather. The funeral service was lovely, Dad would have been proud and we all were able to meet and break bread in memory of a beautiful person.

My message to you would probably be to live life to the fullest, support your loved ones especially in their last moments. It was very challenging at times to follow their wishes such as staying at home because then there was no buffer. We were in the front lines. At an Assisted Living facility there would have been a buffer and you would have been 'notified' of their pending death. At home, you can say you were there, he knew the family was there holding his hand and reassuring him. Simply said, saying 'I love you' is the most beautiful final words that can be shared.

What Now…

To find out more about what the Alzheimer's Disease is, and to find out more about the umbrella of Dementia, begin an online research by browsing for information on: 'What is Alzheimer's' and 'What is Dementia'. Then visit www.alz.org, the Alzheimer's organization website. The Alzheimer's Association (ALZ) is the leading voluntary health organization on Alzheimer's care, support and research. The ALZ organization's mission is to eliminate Alzheimer's disease through the advancement of research; to provide and enhance care and support for all affected; and to reduce the risk of dementia through the promotion of brain health (www.alz.org).

As time went on, at the age of 89, Dad really started to decline as a result of dementia. My lesson learned during this time, is to trust the doctors and the nurses. At the same time, continue to persevere in getting the necessary treatment to make the patient comfortable. There is no reason to suffer – you or them.

Each of the Deli Girls are unique and special. In understanding the effects of the disease on the family and the caretakers is to remember that one cannot catch a break from this disease. All of the caretakers from the Deli Girls, needed help because even though the Deli Girls were Wonder Women, they couldn't do it all! Many discussions were about who can help and how can we pay for the extra help. If you had veteran benefits, help was available. If you had Medicaid, help was available. Sometimes other insurance policies such as Long Term Care insurance had benefits where help was available. What I personally witnessed, was most of us worked for a living, retired with a pension, collected Social Security and paid for Medicare. It wasn't enough to pay for the services and help needed to care for someone with dementia. In Fairfax County, Virginia (2017-2018), the average in-home care by visiting nurses normally averaged $25 per hour with a 4 hour minimum (in the State of Virginia). In my research, the average cost for memory care facilities range from $5,000 to $10,000/month, sometimes more depending on location and client needs (www.agingcare.com, 2019). Most of the Deli Girls had family help, or creatively financed what they could.

In our experience, Dad would sleep all day and it was at night time that he required more care. Again we were blessed, there were three of us kids and we all helped where we could. My greater contribution to my family was to be there to help care for my dad, especially in the last few months when his health was steadily declining.

Mom and Dad were married for 66 years and if Dad lived for one more month, they would have been married officially for 67 years! One marries in "sickness and in health, for richer or for poorer". In this case, 'in sickness' was both exhausting and traumatizing in its own way. Watching a love one struggle to breathe and to lay in discomfort was in itself a struggle. I don't know if I ever accepted his illness or not, but I did find ways to enjoy my time with Dad. He was a pretty happy guy during the times of rest probably because he didn't fully realize what was going on. I believe that to be a blessing – why should he worry about all of that? Don't get me wrong, the disease of dementia has you ask the questions of 'why is this happening?' and 'How long is this going to go on for?' and 'Is Dad suffering?'. I had no answers. The best thing for me to do was to enjoy my time with Dad and do what I could to help in moments of crisis, which were many.

In conclusion, I am 61 years old at the time of this publishing, I am still misplacing my keys, sometimes I have to search for the television remote and yes, I have to make lists. I am very much aware that there is this question looming over me but at this time, I try to stay healthy and plan for the future. More importantly, I learned through my father's journey, to focus on the moment, be happy and enjoy life. My mother was the primary caretaker in caring for my father, her husband, was a hard burden for her to carry. A lot of old resentments and frustrations came up for her with regrets of not pursuing old dreams. It is so important that caretakers find support, find rest and find places of happiness. My mother is an artist. She enjoys oil paintings and to this day, at the age of 92, she continues her artwork. My mother was able to keep sane, keep strong by leaning on her support group, The Deli Girls, and finding enjoyment in her artwork. All we can do is enjoy life, learn from our memories and to live life one day at a time.

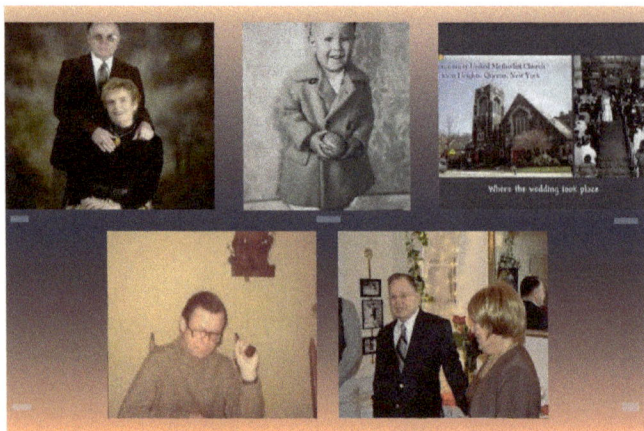

From Left to Right (top row): Mom/Dad 50th anniversary picture; Dad as a little boy; The church they were married in (bottom row): Dad enjoying his pipe; Dad and Mom at their 60th wedding anniversary in 2012

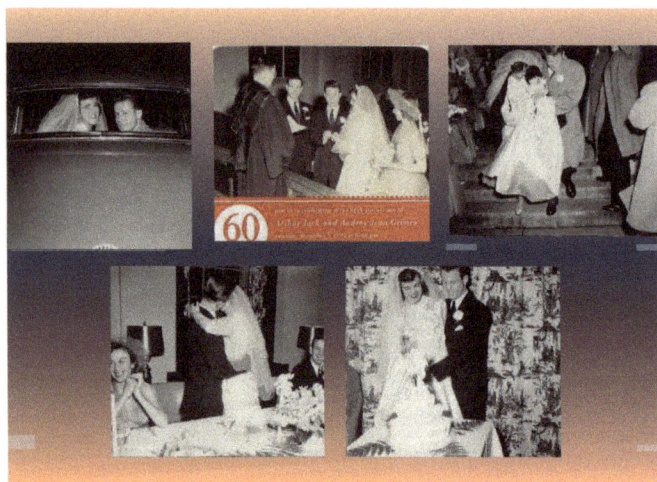

From Left to Right (top row): "Just Married"; 60th Wedding Anniversary Invitation 2012; Leaving the church
(bottom row): Wedding Reception kiss; Wedding Reception cutting the cake.

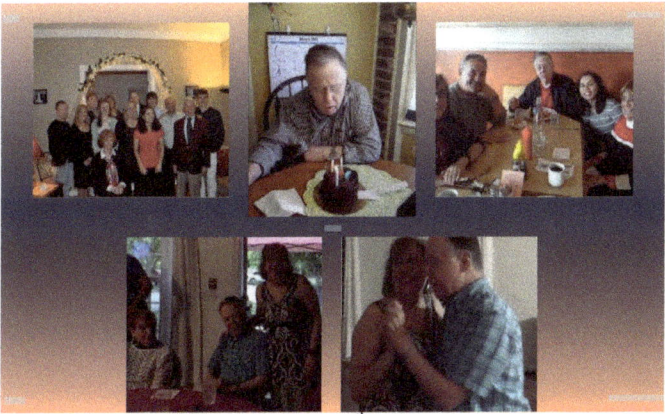

From Left to Right (top row): 2012 60th Anniversary party – the family; Dad at 89 years old; Taking time out for lunch (bottom row): 2015 Graduation party 1) Enjoying the party 2) Enjoying the dance (great dance partner!)

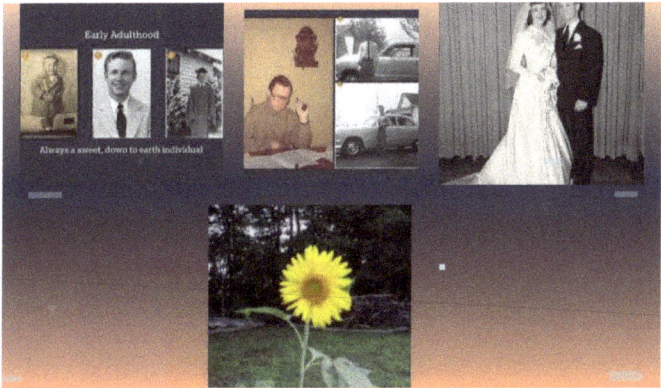

From Left to Right (top row): Young Adult pictures; Dad enjoying his pipe, his car; Wedding picture (1952) (bottom row): This flower is shining and always in our hearts!

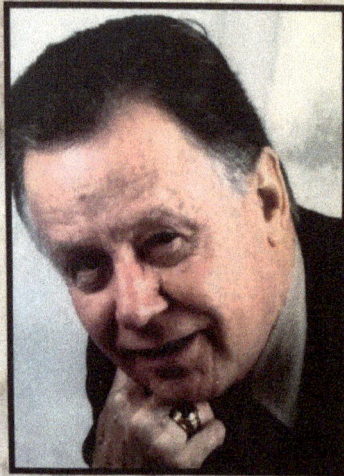

In Memory of

Arthur Jackson "Jack" Grimes

April 4, 1928 – November 23, 2018

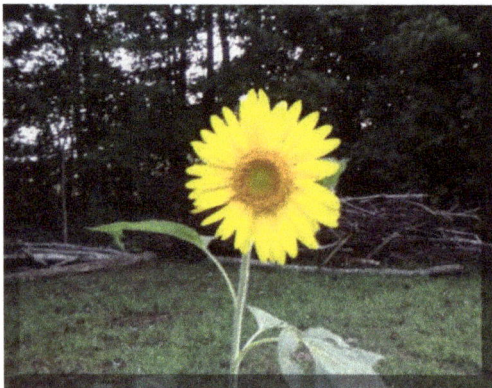

Winds of Change:
Inside the Mind of Alzheimer's
(As written by Greg O'Brien)

"Alzheimer's did not kill his spirit. He lived his life with courage and wisdom."

"...So, Steve adjusted the course when diagnosed with Early Onset Alzheimer's in 2011 at age 59. Sharing the tiller with selfless love and support from his caregiving wife Judy, the couple put retirement plans on hold with storm clouds massing on the horizon and morphed into one—Judy becoming her husband's compass; Steve, her ballast. Alzheimer's is a family disease, one in which the caregiver, the heroes of this disease, must maneuver through the fog, attempting to avoid the flotsam and jetsam of the killer in waiting."

"Steve is now free of the chains," said Judy. "He carried them with grace." (O'Brien, 2018)

Memorialization
Arthur Jack Grimes

Born April 4, 1928 in Macon, Georgia - Died November 23, 2018, at home in Annandale, Virginia surrounded by family. Jack grew up in Macon, Georgia, San Antonio, Texas, then Newport News, Virginia. While in High School, he was awarded a full scholarship to the college of William and Mary, a research University in Williamsburg, Virginia where he received his Bachelor in Science. He then moved to New York City to attend Columbia University where he received his Masters in Public Health Administration. He worked for NPA, the National Pesticides Association until he retired. One of Jack's remarkable strengths is that he lived with Type1 diabetes for 77 years. He received a medal from the Joselin Center for Diabetes for his courageous efforts in living with this disease. Jack was married to Audrey Jean Fenton Grimes since December 6, 1952 for 66 years (December 6, 2018 would have been their 67th anniversary). They have three children Susan (Scott), David, Pamela (John) and have eight very special grand-children (Benjamin, Jeffrey, Caleigh, Brian, Katelyn, Jeffrey, Mark and Jordanka). Jack enjoyed retirement by starting The Professional Group at the George Mason University (Senior professional Consulting) following his attendance at the Lincolnia Senior Center. Jack could be very funny at times and enjoyed being social. We will all miss him as a husband and as a Dad. We were blessed to have him with us as long as we did.

References

Ellison, J. M. (2019). Is Alzheimer's a Genetic Disease? Retrieved from https://www.brightfocus.org/alzheimers/article/alzheimers-genetic-disease?

O'Brien, G. (2018). Winds of Change: Inside the Mind of Alzheimer's. Retrieved from https://www.psychologytoday.com/us/blog/pluto/201804/winds-change-inside-the-mind-alzheimer-s

Reagan, R. (1994). Text of letter written by President Ronald Reagan announcing he has Alzheimer's disease. Retrieved from https://www.reaganlibrary.gov/sreference/reagan-s-letter-announcing-his-alzheimer-s-diagnosis